The Complete Renal Diet Cookbook

An Impeccable Guide with Mouthwatering Recipes to Improve Kidney Function and Live Healthily

EDWARD STEVENS

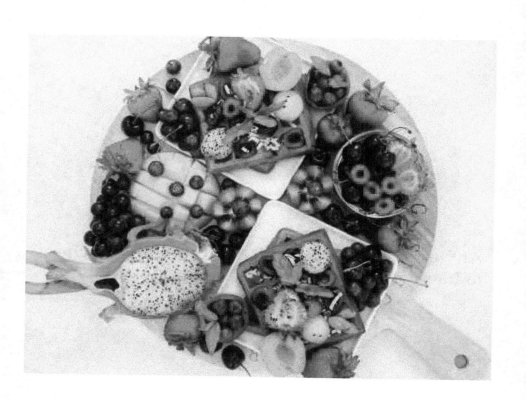

Table of Content

—
4

Additionally, the information in the following pages is intended only for informational purposes and should thus be thought of as universal. As befitting its nature, it is presented without assurance regarding its prolonged validity or interim quality. Trademarks that are mentioned are done without written consent and can in no way be considered an endorsement from the trademark holder.

Introduction

Human health hangs in a complete balance when all of its interconnected bodily mechanisms function properly in perfect sync. Without its major organs working normally, the body soon suffers indelible damage. Kidney malfunction is one such example, and it is not just the entire water balance that is disturbed by the kidney disease, but a number of other diseases also emerge due to this problem.

Kidney diseases are progressive, meaning that they can ultimately lead to permanent kidney damage if left unchecked and uncontrolled. That is why it is essential to control and manage the disease and halt its progress, which can be done through medicinal and natural means. While medicines can guarantee only thirty percent of the cure, a change of lifestyle and diet can prove miraculous with their seventy percent guaranteed results. A kidney-friendly diet and lifestyle not only saves the kidneys from excess minerals, but it also aids medicines to work actively. Treatment without a good diet, hence, proves to be useless. In this renal diet cookbook, we shall bring out the basic facts about kidney diseases, their symptoms, causes, and diagnosis. This preliminary introduction can help the readers understand the problem clearly; then, we shall discuss the role of renal diet and kidney-friendly lifestyle in curbing the diseases. It's not just that the book also contains a range of delicious renal diet recipes, which will guarantee luscious flavors and good health.

Despite their tiny size, the kidneys perform a number of functions, which are vital for the body to be able to function healthily.

These include:

- Filtering excess fluids and waste from the blood.

- Creating the enzyme known as renin, which regulates blood pressure.

- Ensuring bone marrow creates red blood cells.

- Controlling calcium and phosphorus levels through absorption and excretion.

Unfortunately, when kidney disease reaches a chronic stage, these functions start to stop working. However, with the right treatment and lifestyle, it is possible to manage symptoms and continue living well. This is even more applicable in the earlier stages of the disease. Tactlessly, 10% of all adults over the age of 20 will experience some form of kidney disease in their lifetime. There are a variety of different treatments for kidney disease, which depend on the cause of the disease.

According to international stats, kidney (or renal) diseases are affecting around 14% of the adult population. In the US, approx. 661.000 Americans suffer from kidney dysfunction. Out of these patients, 468.000 proceed to dialysis treatment, and the rest have one active kidney transplant.

The high quantities of diabetes and heart illness are also related to kidney dysfunction, and sometimes one condition, for example, diabetes, may prompt the other.

With such a significant number of high rates, possibly the best course of treatment is the contravention of dialysis, making people depend upon clinical and crisis facility meds in any occasion multiple times every week. In this manner, if your kidney has just given a few indications of brokenness, you can forestall dialysis through an eating routine, something that we will talk about in this book.

Chapter 1. The Renal Diet

The Benefits of Renal diet

If you have been diagnosed with kidney dysfunction, a proper diet is necessary for controlling the amount of toxic waste in the bloodstream. When toxic waste piles up in the system along with increased fluid, chronic inflammation occurs, and we have a much higher chance of developing cardiovascular, bone, metabolic, or other health issues.

Since your kidneys can't fully get rid of the waste on their own, which comes from food and drinks, probably the only natural way to help our system is through this diet.

A renal diet is especially useful during the first stages of kidney dysfunction and leads to the following benefits:

● Prevents excess fluid and waste build-up

● prevents the progression of renal dysfunction stages

● Decreases the likelihood of developing other chronic health problems, e.g., heart disorders

● has a mild antioxidant function in the body, which keeps inflammation and inflammatory responses under control.

The benefits mentioned above are noticeable once the patient follows the diet for at least a month and then continuing it for longer periods to avoid the stage where dialysis is needed. The diet's strictness depends on the current stage of renal/kidney disease if, for example, if you are in the 3rd or 4th stage, you should follow a stricter diet and be attentive to the food, which is allowed or prohibited.

Nutrients You Need

Potassium

Potassium is a naturally occurring mineral found in nearly all foods in varying amounts. Our bodies need an amount of potassium to help with muscle activity as well as electrolyte balance and regulation of blood pressure. However, if potassium is in excess within the system and the kidneys can't expel it (due to renal disease), fluid retention and muscle spasms can occur.

Phosphorus

Phosphorus is a trace mineral found in a wide range of foods and especially dairy, meat, and eggs. It acts synergistically with calcium as well as Vitamin D to promote bone health. However, when there is damage in the kidneys, excess amounts of the mineral cannot be taken out, causing bone weakness.

Calories

When being on a renal diet, it is vital to give yourself the right number of calories to fuel your system. The exact number of calories you should consume daily depends on your age, gender, general health status, and stage of renal disease. In most cases, though, there are no strict limitations in the calorie intake, as long as you take them from proper sources that are low in sodium, potassium, and phosphorus. In general, doctors recommend a daily limit between 1800-2100 calories per day to keep weight within the normal range.

Protein

Protein is an essential nutrient that our systems need to develop and generate new connective tissue, e.g., muscles, even during injuries. Protein also helps stop bleeding and supports the immune system to fight infections. A healthy adult with no kidney disease would usually need 40-65 grams of protein per day.

However, in a renal diet, protein consumption is a tricky subject as too much or too little can cause problems. When metabolized by our systems, protein also creates waste, which is typically processed by the kidneys. However, when kidneys are damaged or underperforming, as in the case of kidney disease, that waste will stay in the system. This is why patients in more advanced CKD stages are advised to limit their protein consumption as well.

Fats

Our systems need fats and particularly good fats as a fuel source and for other metabolic cell functions. A diet high in bad or trans fats can significantly increase the chances of developing heart problems, which often occur with kidney disease. This is why most physicians advise their renal patients to follow a diet that contains a decent amount of good fats and a meager amount of Trans (processed) or saturated fat.

Sodium

Sodium is what our bodies need to regulate fluid and electrolyte balance. It also plays a role in normal cell division in the muscles and nervous system. However, in kidney disease, sodium can quickly spike at higher than normal levels, and the kidneys will be unable to expel it, causing fluid accumulation as a side-effect. Those who also suffer from heart problems as well should limit its consumption as it may raise blood pressure.

Carbohydrates

Carbs act as a major and quick fuel source for the body's cells. When we consume carbs, our systems turn them into glucose and then into energy for "feeding" our body cells. Carbs are generally not restricted in the renal diet. Still, some types of carbs contain dietary fiber as well, which helps regulate normal colon function and protect blood vessels from damage.

Dietary Fiber

Fiber is an important element in our system that cannot be properly digested, but plays a key role in the regulation of our bowel movements and blood cell protection. The fiber in the renal diet is generally encouraged as it helps loosen up the stools, relieve constipation and bloating and protect from colon damage. However, many patients don't get enough amounts of dietary fiber per day, as many of them are high in potassium or phosphorus. Fortunately, there are some good dietary fiber sources for CKD patients that have lower amounts of these minerals compared to others.

Vitamins/Minerals

According to medical research, our systems need at least 13 vitamins and minerals to keep our cells fully active and healthy. However, patients with renal disease are more likely to be depleted by water-soluble vitamins like B-complex and Vitamin C as a result of limited fluid consumption. Therefore, supplementation with these vitamins, along with a renal diet program, should help cover any possible vitamin deficiencies. Supplementation of fat-soluble vitamins like vitamins A, K, and E may be avoided as they can quickly build up in the system and turn toxic.

Fluids

When you are in an advanced stage of renal disease, fluid can quickly build-up and lead to problems. While it is important to keep your system well hydrated, you should avoid minerals like potassium and sodium, which can trigger further fluid build-up and cause a host of other symptoms.

Nutrient You Need to Avoid

Salt or sodium is known for being one of the most important ingredients that the renal diet prohibits its use. This ingredient, although simple, can badly and strongly affect your body, especially the kidneys. Any excess of sodium can't be easily filtered because of the failing condition of the kidneys. A large build-up of sodium can cause catastrophic results on your body. Potassium and Phosphorus are also prohibited for kidney patients depending on the stage of kidney disease.

Chapter 2. Kidney disease

What is Kidney Disease?

A kidney disease diagnosis implies that the kidneys are either dysfunctional, under-functioning, or damaged and cannot filter out toxins and metabolic waste on their own. Our systems need our kidneys for a waste filtering process. However, when kidney damage occurs, the system is piled up with damaging waste that cannot expel through other means. As a result, inflammatory responses emerge, and you have a much higher chance of developing chronic and serious health disorders like diabetes or heart failure, which can even be fatal in extreme cases.

There are two main types of kidney disease, based on their cause and time duration:

● A sudden and unexpected kidney damage/acute kidney injury (AKI) as a result of an accident or surgery side effects, which usually lasts for a short period of time.

● Chronic and progressive kidney dysfunction (CKD). As its name suggests, this is a chronic condition with multiple progressive stages that lead ultimately to permanent kidney damage. There are approx. 5 stages of the disorder, and during the last and final stage, the patient will need dialysis or a kidney transplant to survive. This final stage is also known in the medical glossary as End-Stage-Renal Disease (ESRD).

There are higher than normal amounts of a certain protein called Arbutin in the urine during all kidney dysfunction stages, which can be confirmed by urine tests for diagnosing renal disease. This condition is known scientifically as Proteinuria. Doctors may also perform blood tests and/or image screening tests to pinpoint a problem with the kidneys and develop a diagnosis.

Causes of Kidney Disease?

There are many causes of kidney disease, including physical injury or disorders that can damage the kidneys, but the two leading causes of kidney disease are diabetes and high blood pressure. These underlying conditions also put people at risk for developing cardiovascular disease. Early treatment may not only slow down the progression of the disease, but also reduce your risk of developing heart disease or stroke.

Kidney disease can affect anyone at any age. African Americans, Hispanics, and American Indians are at increased risk for kidney failure because these groups have a greater prevalence of diabetes and high blood pressure.

Uncontrolled diabetes is the leading cause of kidney disease. Diabetes can damage the kidneys and cause them to fail.

The second leading cause of kidney disease is high blood pressure, also known as hypertension. One in three Americans is at risk for kidney disease because of hypertension. Although there is no cure for hypertension, certain medications, a low-sodium diet, and physical activity can lower blood pressure.

The kidneys help manage blood pressure, but when blood pressure is high, the heart has to work overtime at pumping blood. High blood pressure can damage the blood vessels in the kidneys, reducing their ability to work efficiently. When the force of blood flow is high, blood vessels start to stretch so the blood can flow more easily. The stretching and scarring weaken the blood vessels throughout the entire body, including the kidneys. When the kidneys' blood vessels are injured, they may not remove the waste and extra fluid from the body, creating a dangerous cycle because the extra fluid in the blood vessels can increase blood pressure even more.

Cardiovascular disease is the leading cause of death in the United States. When kidney disease occurs, that process can be affected, and the risk of developing heart disease becomes greater. Cardiovascular disease is an umbrella term used to describe conditions that may damage the heart and blood vessels, including coronary artery disease, heart attack, heart failure, atherosclerosis, and high blood pressure. Complications from a renal disease may develop and can lead to heart disease.

With diabetes, excess blood sugar remains in the bloodstream. The high blood sugar levels can damage the blood vessels in the kidneys and elsewhere in the body. And since high blood pressure is a complication from diabetes, the extra pressure can weaken the walls of the blood vessels, which can lead to a heart attack or stroke.

Other conditions, such as drug abuse and certain autoimmune diseases, can also cause injury to the kidneys. In fact, every drug we put into our body has to pass through the kidneys for filtration. If the drug is not taken following a healthcare provider's instructions, or if it is an illegal substance such as heroin, cocaine, or ecstasy, it can cause injury to the kidneys by raising the blood pressure, also increasing the risk of a stroke, heart failure, and even death.

An autoimmune disease is one in which the immune system, designed to protect the body from illness, sees the body as an invader and attacks its own systems, including the kidneys. Some forms of lupus, for example, attack the kidneys. Another autoimmune disease that can lead to kidney failure is Goodpasture syndrome, a group of conditions that affect the kidneys and the lungs. The damage to the kidneys from autoimmune diseases can lead to chronic kidney disease and kidney failure.

Symptoms of Kidney Disease?

Some people in the early stages of kidney disease may not even show any symptoms. If you suffer from diabetes or high blood pressure, it is important to manage it early on in order to protect your kidneys. Although kidney failure occurs over the course of many years, you may not show any signs until kidney disease or failure has occurred.

When the kidneys are damaged, wastes and toxins can build up in the body because the kidneys cannot filter them as effectively. Once this buildup begins, you may start to feel sick and experience some of the following symptoms:

- Anemia (low red blood cell count)
- Blood in urine
- Bone pain
- Difficulty concentrating
- Difficulty sleeping
- Dry and itchy skin
- Muscle cramps (especially in the legs)
- Nausea
- Poor appetite
- Swelling in feet and ankles
- Tiredness
- Weakness
- Weight loss

Fortunately, once treatment for kidney disease begins, especially if caught in the early stages, symptoms tend to lessen, and general health will begin to improve.

Diagnosis Tests

Besides identifying the symptoms of kidney disease, there are other better and more accurate ways to confirm the extent of loss of renal function. There are mainly two important diagnostic tests:

1. Urine Test

The urine test clearly states all the renal problems. The urine is the waste product of the kidney. When there is a loss of filtration or any hindrance to the kidneys, the urine sample will indicate it through the number of excretory products present in it. The severe stages of chronic disease show some amount of protein and blood in the urine. Do not rely on self-tests; visit an authentic clinic for these tests.

2. Blood Pressure and Blood Test

Another good way to check for renal disease is to test the blood and its composition. A high amount of creatinine and other waste products in the blood clearly indicates that the kidneys are not functioning properly. Blood pressure can also be indicative of renal disease. When the water balance in the body is disturbed, it may cause high blood pressure. Hypertension can both be the cause and symptom of kidney disease and, therefore, should be taken seriously.

Treatment

The best way to manage CKD is to be an active participant in your treatment program, regardless of your stage of renal disease. Proper treatment involves a combination of working with a healthcare team, adhering to a renal diet, and making healthy lifestyle decisions. These can all have a profoundly positive effect on your kidney disease—especially watching how you eat.

Working with Your Healthcare Team

When you have kidney disease, working in partnership with your healthcare team can be extremely important in your treatment program as well as being personally empowering. Regularly meeting with your physician or healthcare team can arm you with resources and information that help you make informed decisions regarding your treatment needs and provide you with a much-needed opportunity to vent, share information, get advice, and receive support in effectively managing this illness.

Adhering to a Renal Diet

The heart of this book is the renal diet. Sticking to this diet can make a huge difference in your health and vitality. Like any change, following the diet may not be easy at first. Important changes to your diet, particularly early on, can possibly prevent the need for dialysis. These changes include limiting salt, eating a low-protein diet, reducing fat intake, and getting enough calories if you need to lose weight. Be honest with yourself first and foremost—learn what you need, and consider your personal goals and obstacles. Start by making small changes. It is okay to have some slip-ups—we all do. With guidance and support, these small changes will become habits of your promising new lifestyle. In no time, you will begin taking control of your diet and health.

Making Healthy Lifestyle Decisions

Lifestyle choices play a crucial part in our health, especially when it comes to helping regulate kidney disease. Lifestyle choices such as allotting time for physical activity, getting enough sleep, managing weight, reducing stress, and limiting smoking and alcohol will help you take control of your overall health, making it easier to manage your kidney disease. Follow this simple formula: Keep toxins out of your body as much as you can, and build up your immune system with a good balance of exercise, relaxation, and sleep.

Chapter 3. Breakfast

1. Tasty Breakfast Donuts

Preparation Time: 5 minutes

Cooking Time: 5 minutes

Servings: 4

Ingredients:

- 43 grams of cream cheese
- 2 eggs
- 2 tablespoons of almond flour
- 2 tablespoons of Erythritol
- 1 ½ tablespoon of coconut flour
- ½ teaspoon of baking powder
- ½ teaspoon of vanilla extract
- 5 drops of Stevia (liquid form)
- 2 strips bacon, fried until crispy

Directions:

1. Rub coconut oil over the donut maker and turn it on.
2. Pulse all the ingredients except bacon in a blender or food processor until smooth (should take around 1 minute).
3. Pour batter into donut maker, leaving 1/10 in each round for rising.
4. Leave for 3 minutes before flipping each donut. Leave for another 2 minutes or until the fork comes out clean when piercing them.
5. Take donuts out and let cool.

6. Repeat steps 1-5 until all batter is used.

7. Crumble bacon into bits and use to top donuts.

Nutrition:

- Calories: 60
- Fat: 5g
- Carbs: 1g
- Fiber: 0g
- Protein: 3g

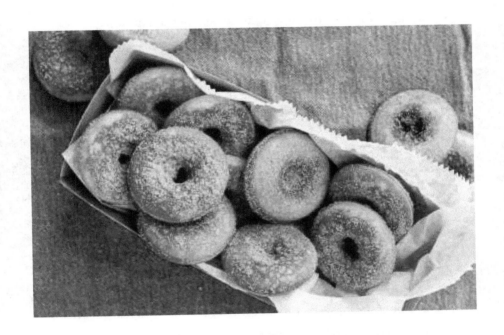

2. Cheesy Spicy Bacon Bowls

Preparation Time: 10 minutes

Cooking Time: 22 minutes

Servings: 12

Ingredients:

- 6 strips of Bacon, pan-fried until cooked but still malleable
- 4 eggs
- 60 grams of cheddar cheese
- 40 grams of cream cheese, grated
- 2 Jalapenos, sliced and seeds removed
- 2 tablespoons of coconut oil
- ¼ teaspoon of onion powder
- ¼ teaspoon of garlic powder
- Dash of salt and pepper

Directions:

1. Preheat oven to 375 °F.
2. In a bowl, beat together the eggs, cream cheese, jalapenos (minus 6 slices), coconut oil, onion powder, garlic powder, and salt and pepper.
3. Using leftover bacon grease on a muffin tray, rubbing it into each insert. Place bacon-wrapped inside the parameters of each insert.
4. Pour beaten mixture halfway up each bacon bowl.
5. Garnish each bacon bowl with cheese and leftover jalapeno slices (placing one on top of each).

6. Leave in the oven for about 22 minutes, or until the egg is thoroughly cooked and cheese is bubbly.

7. Remove from oven and let cool until edible.

8. Enjoy!

Nutrition:

- Calories: 259
- Fat: 24g
- Carbs: 1g
- Fiber: 0g
- Protein: 10g

3. Goat Cheese Zucchini Kale Quiche

Preparation Time: 35 minutes

Cooking Time: 1 hour 10 minutes

Servings: 4

Ingredients:

- 4 large eggs
- 8 ounces of fresh zucchini, sliced
- 10 ounces of kale
- 3 garlic cloves (minced)
- 1 cup of soy milk
- 1 ounce of goat cheese
- 1cup of grated parmesan
- 1cup of shredded cheddar cheese
- 2 teaspoons of olive oil
- Salt & pepper, to taste

Directions:

1. Preheat oven to 350°F.
2. Heat 1 tsp. of olive oil in a saucepan over medium-high heat. Sauté garlic for 1 minute until flavored.
3. Add the zucchini and cook for another 5-7 minutes until soft.
4. Beat the eggs, and then add a little milk and Parmesan cheese.
5. Meanwhile, heat the remaining olive oil in another saucepan and add the cabbage. Cover and cook for 5 minutes until dry.
6. Slightly grease a baking dish with cooking spray and spread the kale leaves across the bottom. Add the zucchini and top with goat cheese.

7. Pour the egg, milk, and parmesan mixture evenly over the other ingredients. Top with cheddar cheese.
8. Bake for 50–60 minutes until golden brown. Check the center of the quiche; it should have a solid consistency.
9. Let chill for a few minutes before serving.

Nutrition:

- Total Carbohydrates: 15g
- Dietary Fiber: 2g
- Net Carbs: 13g
- Protein: 19g
- Total Fat: 18g
- Calories: 290

4. Cream Cheese Egg Breakfast

Preparation Time: 5 minutes

Cooking Time: 5 minutes

Servings: 4

Ingredients:

- 2 eggs, beaten
- 1 tablespoon of butter
- 2 tablespoons of soft cream cheese with chives

Directions:

1. Melt the butter in a small skillet.
2. Add the eggs and cream cheese.
3. Stir and cook to desired doneness.

Nutrition:

- Calories: 341
- Fat: 31g
- Protein: 15g
- Carbohydrate: 0g
- Dietary Fiber: 3g

5. Avocado Red Peppers Roasted Scrambled Eggs

Preparation Time: 10 minutes

Cooking Time: 12 minutes

Servings: 3

Ingredients:

- 1/2 tablespoon of butter
- 2 Eggs
- 1/2 roasted red pepper, about 1 1/2 ounces
- 1/2 small avocado, coarsely chopped, about 2 1/4 ounces
- Salt, to taste

Directions:

1. In a nonstick skillet, heat the butter over medium heat. Break the eggs into the pan and break the yolks with a spoon. Sprinkle with a little salt.
2. Stir to stir and continue stirring until the eggs start to come out. Quickly add the bell peppers and avocado.
3. Cook and stir until the eggs suit your taste. Adjust the seasoning, if necessary.

Nutrition:

- Calories: 317
- Fat: 26g
- Protein: 14g

- Dietary Fiber: 5g
- Net Carbs: 4g

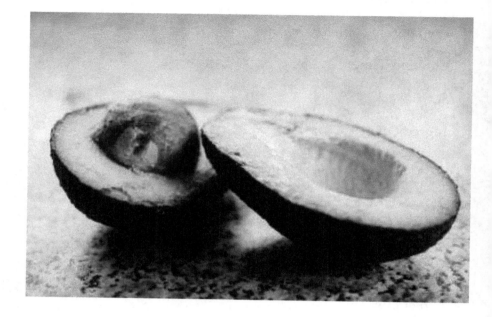

6. Mushroom Quickie Scramble

Preparation Time: 10 minutes

Cooking Time: 10 minutes

Servings: 4

Ingredients:

- 3 small-sized eggs, whisked
- 4 pcs. of bella mushrooms
- ½ cup of spinach
- ¼ cup of red bell peppers
- 2 deli ham slices
- 1 tablespoon of ghee or coconut oil
- Salt & pepper to taste

Directions:

1. Chop the ham and veggies.
2. Put half a tbsp. of butter in a frying pan and heat until melted.
3. Sauté the ham and vegetables in a frying pan, then set aside.
4. Get a new frying pan and heat the remaining butter.
5. Add the whisked eggs into the second pan while stirring continuously to avoid overcooking.
6. When the eggs are done, sprinkle with salt & pepper to taste.
7. Add the ham and veggies to the pan with the eggs.
8. Mix well.
9. Remove from burner and transfer to a plate.
10. Serve and enjoy.

Nutrition:

- Calories: 350
- Total Fat: 29 g
- Protein: 21 g
- Total Carbs: 5 g

7. Coconut Coffee and Ghee

Preparation Time: 10 minutes

Cooking Time: 10 minutes

Servings: 5

Ingredients:

- ½ Tbsp. of coconut oil
- ½ Tbsp. of ghee
- 1 to 2 cups of preferred coffee (or rooibos or black tea, if preferred)
- 1 Tbsp. of coconut or almond milk

Directions:

1. Place the almond (or coconut) milk, coconut oil, ghee, and coffee in a blender (or milk frother).
2. Mix for around 10 seconds or until the coffee turns creamy and foamy.
3. Pour contents into a coffee cup.
4. Serve immediately and enjoy.

Nutrition:

- Calories: 150
- Total Fat: 15 g
- Protein: 0 g
- Total Carbs: 0 g
- Net Carbs: 0 g

8. Yummy Veggie Waffles

Preparation Time: 10 minutes

Cooking Time: 9 minutes

Servings: 3

Ingredients:

- 3 cups of raw cauliflower, grated
- 1 cup of cheddar cheese
- 1 cup of mozzarella cheese
- ½ cup of parmesan
- 1/3 cup of chives, finely sliced
- 6 eggs
- 1 teaspoon of garlic powder
- 1 teaspoon of onion powder
- ½ teaspoon of chili flakes
- Dash of salt and pepper

Directions:

1. Turn the waffle maker on.
2. In a bowl, mix all the listed ingredients very well until incorporated.
3. Once the waffle maker is hot, distribute the waffle mixture into the insert.
4. Let cook for about 9 minutes, flipping at 6 minutes.
5. Remove from waffle maker and set aside.
6. Repeat the previous steps with the rest of the batter until gone (should come out to 4 waffles)
7. Serve and enjoy!

Nutrition:

- Calories: 390
- Fat: 28g
- Carbs: 6g
- Fiber: 2g
- Protein: 30g

9. Omega 3 Breakfast Shake

Preparation Time: 5 minutes

Cooking Time: 5 minutes

Servings: 2

Ingredients:

- 1 cup of vanilla almond milk (unsweetened)
- 2 tablespoons of blueberries
- 1 ½ tablespoon of flaxseed meal
- 1 tablespoon of MCT Oil
- ¾ tablespoon of banana extract
- ½ tablespoon of chia seeds
- 5 Drops of Stevia (liquid form)
- 1/8 tablespoon of Xanthan gum

Directions:

1. In a blender, pulse vanilla almond milk, banana extract, Stevia, and 3 ice cubes.
2. When smooth, add blueberries and pulse.
3. Once blueberries are thoroughly incorporated, add flaxseed meal and chia seeds.
4. Let sit for 5 minutes.
5. After 5 minutes, pulse again until all ingredients are nicely distributed. Serve and enjoy.

Nutrition:

- Calories: 264
- Fats: 25g
- Carbs: 7g
- Protein: 4g

10. Delicious Pesto Pork Chops

Prep:

20 mins

Cook:

1 hr 40 mins

Total:

2 hrs

Servings:

6

Yield:

6 servings

Ingredients

6 pork chops
1 teaspoon garlic powder
1 teaspoon seasoned salt, or to taste
2 eggs
¼ cup all-purpose flour
2 cups Italian-style seasoned bread crumbs
¼ cup olive oil
1 (10.75 ounce) can condensed cream of chicken soup
½ cup milk
3 tablespoons pesto

Directions

1

Preheat oven to 350 degrees F (175 degrees C).

2

Season pork chops with garlic powder and seasoned salt.

3

Beat eggs in a bowl until smooth. Pour flour into a separate shallow bowl and bread crumbs into a third bowl.

4

Gently press seasoned pork chops into the flour to coat and shake to remove excess flour. Dip into the beaten egg, then press into bread crumbs. Gently toss between your hands so any bread crumbs that haven't stuck can fall away. Place the breaded chops onto a plate while breading the rest; do not stack.

5

Heat olive oil in a skillet over medium-high heat.

6

Cook pork chops in hot oil until the bread crumb coating is well browned, about 5 minutes per side; transfer to a baking dish. Cover baking dish with aluminum foil.

7

Bake chops in preheated oven for 1 hour. Whisk cream of chicken soup, milk, and pesto together in a bowl; pour over the pork chops. Replace foil and continue baking another 30 minutes.

Nutritions
Per Serving: 531 calories; protein 35.1g; carbohydrates 36.5g; fat 26.6g; cholesterol 129.2mg; sodium 1251.1mg.

11. Fantastic Angel Eggs

Prep:

20 mins

Cook:

15 mins

Additional:

10 mins

Total:

45 mins

Servings:

24

Yield:

24 appetizers

Ingredients

6 tablespoons creamy salad dressing (such as Miracle Whip®)
2 tablespoons sweet pickle relish
12 eggs
1/2 cup ranch dressing
1 tablespoon prepared yellow mustard
¼ teaspoon celery seed
ground black pepper to taste
¼ teaspoon paprika, for garnish

Directions

1

Place eggs into a large saucepan, cover with water, and bring to a boil.

2

Cook for 15 minutes, and cool the eggs under a stream of cold water in the sink, 10 to 15 minutes.

3

Peel the eggs and slice in half lengthwise.

4

Scoop the egg yolks into a bowl, and mash them with a fork.

5

Mix in the ranch dressing, creamy salad dressing, pickle relish, yellow mustard, celery seed, and black pepper until thoroughly combined.

6

Spoon the filling into the egg white halves.

7

Sprinkle each egg half with a pinch of paprika.

Nutritions
Per Serving: fat 4.8g; cholesterol 94.8mg; sodium 105.6mg.

12. Tasty Pepperoni Omelet

Prep:

15 mins

Cook:

10 mins

Total:

25 mins

Servings:

2

Yield:

2 omelets

Ingredients

½ can pizza sauce
1 pinch dried oregano, or to taste
salt and ground black pepper to taste
1 package sliced pepperoni, or to taste
½ tomato, diced
¼ cup diced onion
1 tablespoon olive oil, or as needed
4 eggs, beaten
¼ cup diced mushrooms
2 tablespoons diced olives

Directions

1

Mix pizza sauce, pepperoni, tomato, onion, mushrooms, olives, oregano, salt, and pepper together in a bowl.

2

Heat oil in a skillet over medium heat. Pour eggs into the hot oil and cook until set, about 5 minutes. Pour pizza sauce mixture over eggs and cook until firm enough to fold 1 side of eggs over the filling creating an omelet, 5 to 10 minutes more.

Nutritions

Per Serving: 418 calories; protein 21.6g; carbohydrates 14.7g; fat 30.2g; cholesterol 401.8mg; sodium 1291.8mg.

Chapter 4. LUNCH

13. Cauliflower Rice

Preparation Time: 10 minutes

Cooking Time: 10 minutes

Servings: 4

Ingredients:

- 1 head cauliflower, sliced into florets
- 1 tablespoon of butter
- Black pepper to taste
- 1/4 teaspoon of garlic powder
- 1/4 teaspoon of herb seasoning blend

Direction:

1. Put cauliflower florets in a food processor.
2. Pulse until consistency is similar to grain.
3. In a pan over medium heat, melt the butter and add the spices.
4. Toss cauliflower rice and cook for 10 minutes.
5. Fluff using a fork before serving.

Nutrition:

- Calories: 47
- Protein: 1g
- Carbohydrates: 4g
- Sodium: 43mg

- Potassium: 206mg
- Phosphorus: 31mg
- Calcium: 16mg

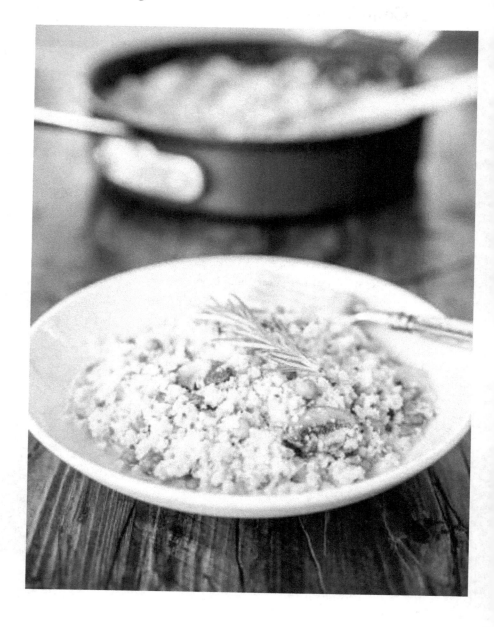

14.Chicken Pineapple Curry

Preparation Time: 40 Minutes

Cooking Time: 3 hours 10 minutes

Servings: 6

Ingredients:

- 1 1/2 lbs. of chicken thighs, boneless, skinless
- 1/2 teaspoon of black pepper
- 1/2 teaspoon of garlic powder
- 2 tablespoons of olive oil
- 20 oz. of canned pineapple
- 2 tablespoons of brown Swerve
- 2 tablespoons of soy sauce
- 1/2 teaspoon of Tabasco sauce
- 2 tablespoons of cornstarch
- 3 tablespoons of water

Direction:

1. Begin by seasoning the chicken thighs with garlic powder and black pepper.
2. Set a suitable skillet over medium-high heat and add the oil to heat.
3. Add the boneless chicken to the skillet and cook for 3 minutes per side.
4. Transfer this seared chicken to a slow cooker, greased with cooking spray.
5. Add 1 cup of the pineapple juice, Swerve, 1 cup of pineapple, tabasco sauce, and soy sauce to a slow cooker.

6. Cover the chicken-pineapple mixture and cook for 3 hours on low heat.

7. Transfer the chicken to the serving plates.

8. Mix the cornstarch with water in a small bowl and pour it into the pineapple curry.

9. Stir and cook this sauce for 2 minutes on high heat until it thickens.

10. Pour this sauce over the chicken and garnish with green onions. Serve warm.

Nutrition:

- Calories: 256
- Fat: 10.4g
- Cholesterol: 67mg
- Sodium: 371mg
- Protein: 22.8g
- Phosphorous: 107mg
- Potassium: 308mg

15.Baked Pork Chops

Preparation Time: 20 Minutes

Cooking Time: 40minutes

Servings: 6

Ingredients:

- 1/2 cup of flour
- 1 large egg
- 1/4 cup of water
- 3/4 cup of breadcrumbs
- 6 (3 1/2 oz.) of pork chops
- 2 tablespoons of butter, unsalted
- 1 teaspoon of paprika

Direction:

1. Begin by switching the oven to 350 °F to preheat.
2. Mix and spread the flour on a shallow plate.
3. Whisk the egg with water in another shallow bowl.
4. Spread the breadcrumbs on a separate plate.
5. Firstly, coat the pork with flour, then dip in the egg mix and then in the crumbs.
6. Grease a baking sheet and place the chops in it.
7. Drizzle the pepper on top and bake for 40 minutes.
8. Serve.

Nutrition:

- Calories: 221

- Sodium: 135mg
- Carbohydrate: 11.9g
- Protein: 24.7g
- Phosphorous: 299mg
- Potassium: 391mg

16. Lasagna Rolls in Marinara Sauce

Preparation Time: 15 Minutes

Cooking Time: 30 minutes

Servings: 9

Ingredients:

- ¼ tsp. of crushed red pepper
- ¼ tsp. of salt
- ½ cup of shredded mozzarella cheese
- ½ cups of parmesan cheese, shredded
- 1 14-oz. of package tofu, cubed
- 1 25-oz. of a can of low-sodium marinara sauce
- 1 tbsp. of extra virgin olive oil
- 12 whole of wheat lasagna noodles
- 2 tbsp. of Kalamata olives, chopped
- 3 cloves minced garlic
- 3 cups of spinach, chopped

Directions:

1. Put enough water on a large pot and cook the lasagna noodles according to the package. Drain, rinse, and set aside until ready to use. In a large skillet, sauté garlic over medium heat for 20 seconds. Add the tofu and spinach and cook until the spinach wilts. Transfer this mixture to a bowl and add parmesan olives, salt, red pepper, and 2/3 cup of the marinara sauce.
2. In a pan, spread a cup of marinara sauce on the bottom. To make the rolls, place noodle on a surface and spread ¼ cup of the tofu filling.

Roll up and place it on the pan with the marinara sauce. Do this procedure until all lasagna noodles are rolled.

3. Place the pan over high heat and bring to a simmer. Reduce the heat to medium and let it cook for three more minutes. Sprinkle mozzarella cheese and let the cheese melt for two minutes. Serve hot.

Nutrition:

- Calories: 600
- Carbs: 65g
- Protein: 36g
- Phosphorus: 627mg
- Potassium: 914mg
- Sodium: 1194mg

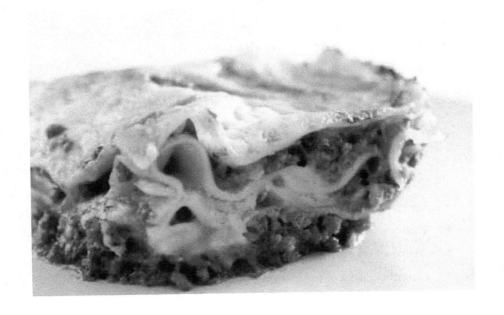

17. Chicken Curry

Preparation Time: 10 Minutes

Cooking Time: 9 Hours

Servings: 5

Ingredients:

- 2 to 3 boneless chicken breasts
- ¼ cup of chopped green onions
- 1 can of 4 oz. of diced green chili peppers
- 2 teaspoons of minced garlic
- 1 and 1/2 teaspoons of curry powder
- 1 teaspoon of chili Powder
- 1 teaspoon of cumin
- ½ teaspoon of cinnamon
- 1 teaspoon of lime juice
- 1 and 1/2 cups of water
- 1 can or 7 oz. of coconut milk
- 2 cups of white cooked rice
- Chopped cilantro, for garnish

Direction:

1. Combine the green onion with the chicken, the green chili peppers, the garlic, the curry powder, the chili powder, the cumin, the cinnamon, the lime juice, and the water in the bottom of a 6-qt slow cooker.

2. Cover the slow cooker with a lid and cook your ingredients on Low for about 7 to 9 hours.

3. After the cooking time ends up, shred the chicken with the help of a fork.
4. Add in the coconut milk and cook on High for about 15 minutes.
5. Top the chicken with cilantro; then serve your dish with rice.
6. Enjoy your lunch!

Nutrition:

- Calories: 254
- Fats: 18g
- Carbs: 6g
- Fiber: 1.6g
- Potassium: 370mg
- Sodium: 240mg
- Phosphorous: 114mg
- Protein 17g

18.Steak with Onion

Preparation Time: 5 Minutes

Cooking Time: 60 Minutes

Servings: 7-8

Ingredients:

- ¼ cup of white flour
- 1/8 Teaspoon of ground black pepper
- 1 and ½ pounds of round steak of ¾ inch of thickness each
- 2 tablespoons of oil
- 1 cup of water
- 1 tablespoon of vinegar
- 1 Minced garlic clove
- 1 to 2 bay leaves
- ¼ teaspoon of crushed dried thyme
- 3 Sliced medium onions

Directions:

1. Cut the steak into about 7 to 8 equal Servings. Combine the flour and the pepper, then pound the Ingredients all together into the meat. Heat the oil in a large skillet over medium-high heat and brown the meat on both its sides.
2. Remove the meat from the skillet and set it aside Combine the water with the vinegar, the garlic, the bay leaf, and the thyme in the skillet; then bring the mixture to a boil.
3. Place the meat in the mixture and cover it with onion slices.
4. Cover your ingredients and let simmer for about 55 to 60 minutes.

5. Serve and enjoy your lunch!

Nutrition:

- Calories: 286
- Fats: 18g
- Carbs: 12g
- Fiber: 2.25g
- Potassium: 368mg
- Sodium: 45mg
- Phosphorous: 180mg
- Protein: 19g

19.Shrimp Scampi

Preparation Time: 4 Minutes

Cooking Time: 8 Minutes

Servings: 3

Ingredients:

- 1 tablespoon of olive oil
- 1 minced garlic clove
- ½ pound of cleaned and peeled shrimp
- ¼ cup of dry white wine
- 1 tablespoon of lemon juice
- ½ teaspoon of basil
- 1 tablespoon of chopped fresh parsley
- 4 oz. of dry linguini

Directions:

1. Heat the oil in a large non-stick skillet; then add the garlic and the shrimp and cook while stirring for about 4 minutes.
2. Add the wine, the lemon juice, the basil, and the parsley.
3. Cook for about 5 minutes longer; then boil the linguini in unsalted water for a few minutes.
4. Drain the linguini, then top it with the shrimp.
5. Serve and enjoy your lunch!

Nutrition:

- Calories: 340
- Fats: 26g
- Carbs: 11.3g
- Fiber: 2.1g
- Potassium: 189mg
- Sodium: 85mg
- Phosphorous: 167mg
- Protein: 15g

20.   Chicken Paella

Preparation Time: 5 Minutes

Cooking Time: 10 Minutes

Servings: 8

Ingredients:

- ½ pound of skinned, boned, and cut into pieces chicken breasts
- 1/4 cup of water
- 1 can of 10-1/2 oz. of low-sodium chicken broth
- ½ pound of peeled and cleaned medium-size shrimp
- 1/2 cup of frozen green pepper
- 1/3 cup of chopped red bell
- 1/3 cup of thinly sliced green onion
- 2 minced garlic cloves
- 1/4 teaspoon of pepper
- 1 dash of ground saffron
- 1 cup of uncooked instant white rice

Direction:

1. Combine the first 3 ingredients in a medium casserole, cover it with a lid, then microwave it for about 4 minutes.
2. Stir in the shrimp and the following 6 ingredients; then cover and microwave the shrimp on high heat for about 3 and ½ minutes.
3. Stir in the rice, then cover and set aside for about 5 minutes.
4. Serve and enjoy your paella!

Nutrition:

- Calories: 236
- Fats: 11g
- Carbs: 6g
- Fiber: 1.2g
- Potassium: 178mg
- Sodium: 83mg
- Phosphorous: 144mg
- Protein: 28g

21.Beef Kabobs with Pepper

Preparation Time: 5 Minutes

Cooking Time: 10 Minutes

Servings: 8

Ingredients:

- 1 Pound of beef sirloin
- ½ cup of vinegar
- 2 tbsp. of salad oil
- 1 medium chopped onion
- 2 tbsp. of chopped fresh parsley
- ¼ tsp. of black pepper
- 2 Cut into strips green peppers

Directions:

1. Trim the fat from the meat, then cut it into cubes of 1 and ½ inches each.
2. Mix the vinegar, the oil, the onion, the parsley, and the pepper in a bowl.
3. Place the meat in the marinade and set it aside for about 2 hours; make sure to stir from time to time.
4. Remove the meat from the marinade and alternate it on skewers instead with green pepper.
5. Brush the pepper with the marinade and broil for about 10 minutes 4 inches from the heat.
6. Serve and enjoy your kabobs.

Nutrition:

- Calories: 357
- Fats: 24g
- Carbs: 9g
- Fiber: 2.3g
- Potassium: 250mg
- Sodium: 60mg
- Phosphorous: 217mg
- Protein: 26g

22. Chicken, Corn and Peppers

Preparation Time: 5 minutes

Cooking Time: 1 hour

Servings: 4

Ingredients:

- 2 pounds chicken breast, skinless, boneless, and cubed
- 2 tablespoons of olive oil
- 2 garlic cloves, minced
- 1 red onion, chopped
- 2 red bell peppers, chopped
- ¼ teaspoon of cumin, ground
- 2 cups of corn
- ½ cup of chicken stock
- 1 teaspoon of chili powder
- ¼ cup of cilantro, chopped

Directions:

1. Heat up a pot with the oil over medium-high heat, add the chicken, and brown for 4 minutes on each side.
2. Add the onion and the garlic and sauté for 5 minutes more.
3. Add the rest of the ingredients, stir, bring to a simmer over medium heat, and cook for 45 minutes.
4. Divide into bowls and serve.

Nutrition:

- Calories: 332

- Fat: 16.1
- Fiber: 8.4
- Carbs: 25.4
- Protein: 17.4

23.   Shrimp Quesadilla

Prep:

15 mins

Cook:

1 hr

Total:

1 hr 15 mins

Servings:

6

Yield:

6 quesadillas

Ingredients

2 tablespoons vegetable oil
1 onion, sliced
1 red bell pepper, sliced
1 green bell pepper, sliced
1 teaspoon salt
1 teaspoon ground cumin
1 teaspoon chili powder
1 pound uncooked medium shrimp, peeled and deveined
1 jalapeno pepper, seeded and minced
1 lime, juiced
1 teaspoon vegetable oil, or as needed
6 large flour tortillas
3 cups shredded Mexican cheese blend, divided

Directions

1

Heat 2 tablespoons vegetable oil in a large skillet over medium-high heat. Cook and stir onion, red bell pepper, and green bell pepper in the hot oil, stirring frequently, until onion is translucent and peppers are soft, 6 to 8 minutes.

2

Stir salt, cumin, and chili powder into onion and bell peppers.

3

Stir shrimp into onion and bell peppers and cook until shrimp are opaque and no longer pink in the center, 3 to 5 minutes.

4

Remove skillet from heat; stir jalapeno pepper and lime juice into shrimp mixture.

5

Heat a skillet over medium heat and brush with about 1 teaspoon vegetable oil.

6

Place a tortilla in the hot oil. Spoon about 1/6 shrimp filling and 1/2 cup Mexican cheese blend on one side of tortilla. Fold tortilla in half.

7

Cook until bottom of tortilla is lightly browned, about 5 minutes; flip and cook other side until lightly browned, 3 to 5 minutes. Repeat with remaining tortillas and filling.

Nutritions
Per Serving: 753 calories; protein 37.9g; carbohydrates 67.8g; fat 36.9g; cholesterol 179.7mg; sodium 1788.4mg.

24.   Almond Chicken

Prep:

30 mins

Cook:

40 mins

Total:

1 hr 10 mins

Servings:

10

Yield:

10 servings

Ingredients

1 (10.5 ounce) can condensed cream of chicken soup
1 (10.5 ounce) can chicken broth
4 cups cooked diced chicken
2 cups water chestnuts, drained (Optional)
2 teaspoons lemon juice
1 ½ cups mayonnaise
2 cups chopped celery
1 small onion, chopped
2 teaspoons salt
2 cups cooked rice
½ cup butter
1 ½ cups crushed buttery round crackers
1 cup sliced almonds
1 cup shredded Colby cheese

Directions

1

Preheat oven to 350 degrees F (175 degrees C).

2

In a large pan over medium heat, stir together cream of chicken soup and water (or broth). Stir in chicken, chestnuts, lemon juice, and mayonnaise. Stir in celery, onion, salt, and rice. Combine well, then pour into a casserole dish.

3

Melt butter in a skillet over medium heat. Pour in crushed crackers, and stir to coat with butter. Pour crackers over the top of casserole. Then sprinkle almonds and shredded cheese over the top.

4

Bake in preheated oven until cheese is melted, about 30 minutes.

Nutritions

Per Serving: 698 calories; protein 25g; carbohydrates 27.7g; fat 54.8g; cholesterol 94.6mg; sodium 1305.1mg.

25.   Platter-O-Brussels

Prep:

45 mins

Total:

45 mins

Servings:

20

Yield:

1 party platter

Ingredients

2 heads iceberg lettuce
1 tablespoon garlic powder
1 tablespoon dried oregano
1 (8 ounce) bottle Italian-style salad dressing
1 pound thinly sliced cooked ham
2 ½ pounds sliced provolone cheese
½ pound Genoa salami, thinly sliced
¼ pound Capacola sausage, sliced
¼ pound pepperoni sausage, sliced
¼ pound prosciutto, thinly sliced
¼ pound thinly sliced roast beef
1 cup fresh mushrooms
1 (6 ounce) can marinated artichoke hearts
1 (7 ounce) jar roasted red peppers
1 (6 ounce) can sliced black olives
¾ cup sliced pepperoncini peppers
1 (5 ounce) jar sliced pimento-stuffed green olives
½ cup crumbled Gorgonzola cheese
½ pound mozzarella cheese, sliced
¼ cup grated Parmesan cheese

Directions

1

Remove large outer leaves from the heads of lettuce. Arrange approximately 1/3 in a layer on a large serving platter. Sprinkle with 1/3 garlic powder, 1/3 crushed oregano and desired amount of Italian-style salad dressing. Layer with cooked ham and Provolone cheese.

2

Layer Provolone cheese with another 1/3 of the lettuce leaves, 1/3 garlic powder, 1/3 crushed oregano, desired amount of Italian-style salad dressing, Genoa salami and Capacola sausage.

3

Repeat layering with remaining lettuce, garlic powder, crushed oregano, Italian-style salad dressing, pepperoni sausage, prosciutto and roast beef.

4

Layer with mushrooms, marinated artichoke hearts, roasted red peppers, black olives, pepperoncini and pimento-stuffed green olives. Sprinkle with more Italian-style salad dressing, as desired.

5

Top with Gorgonzola cheese, mozzarella cheese and Parmesan cheese. Cover and chill in the refrigerator until serving.

Nutritions

Per Serving: 503 calories; protein 31.3g; carbohydrates 7.4g; fat 39g; cholesterol 93.7mg; sodium 2208.7mg.

Chapter 5. DINNER

26. Baked Fennel & Garlic Sea Bass

Preparation Time: 5 minutes

Cooking Time: 15 minutes

Servings: 2

Ingredients:

- 1 lemon
- ½ sliced fennel bulb
- 6 oz. of sea bass fillets
- 1 tsp. of black pepper
- 2 garlic cloves

Direction:

1. Preheat the oven to 375°F/Gas Mark 5.
2. Sprinkle black pepper over the Sea Bass.
3. Slice the fennel bulb and garlic cloves.
4. Add 1 salmon fillet and half the fennel and garlic to one sheet of baking paper or tin foil.
5. Squeeze in 1/2 lemon juices.
6. Repeat for the other fillet.
7. Fold and add to the oven for 12-15 minutes or until fish is thoroughly cooked through.
8. Meanwhile, add boiling water to your couscous, cover, and allow to steam.
9. Serve with your choice of rice or salad.

Nutrition:

- Calories: 221
- Protein: 14 g
- Carbs: 3 g
- Fat: 2 g
- Sodium (Na): 119 mg
- Potassium (K): 398 mg
- Phosphorus: 149 mg

27. Lemon, Garlic & Cilantro Tuna and Rice

Preparation Time: 5 minutes

Cooking Time: 0 minutes

Servings: 2

Ingredients:

- ½ cup of arugula
- 1 tbsp. of extra virgin olive oil
- 1 cup of cooked rice
- 1 tsp. of black pepper
- ¼ finely diced red onion
- 1 juiced lemon
- 3 oz. of canned tuna
- 2 tbsp. of Chopped fresh cilantro

Directions:

1. Mix the olive oil, pepper, cilantro, and red onion in a bowl.
2. Stir in the tuna, cover, and leave in the fridge for as long as possible (if you can) or serve immediately.
3. When ready to eat, serve up with the cooked rice and arugula!

Nutrition:

- Calories: 221
- Protein: 11 g
- Carbs: 26 g

- Fat: 7 g
- Sodium (Na): 143 mg
- Potassium (K): 197 mg
- Phosphorus: 182 mg

28.   Cod & Green Bean Risotto

Preparation Time: 4 minutes

Cooking Time: 40 minutes

Servings: 2

Ingredients:

- ½ cup of arugula
- 1 finely diced white onion
- 4 oz. of cod fillet
- 1 cup of white rice
- 2 lemon wedges
- 1 cup of boiling water
- ¼ tsp. of black pepper
- 1 cup of low sodium chicken broth
- 1 tbsp. of extra virgin olive oil
- ½ cup of green beans

Direction:

1. Heat the oil in a large pan on medium heat. Sauté the chopped onion for 5 minutes until soft before adding in the rice and stirring for 1-2 minutes.
2. Combine the broth with boiling water.
3. Add half of the liquid to the pan and stir slowly.
4. Slowly add the rest of the liquid whilst continuously stirring for up to 20-30 minutes.
5. Stir in the green beans to the risotto.
6. Place the fish on top of the rice, cover, and steam for 10 minutes.

7. Ensure the water does not dry out and keep topping up until the rice is cooked thoroughly.
8. Use your fork to break up the fish fillets and stir into the rice.
9. Sprinkle with freshly ground pepper to serve and a squeeze of fresh lemon.
10. Garnish with the lemon wedges and serve with the arugula.

Nutrition:

- Calories: 221
- Protein: 12 g
- Carbs: 29 g
- Fat: 8 g
- Sodium (Na): 398 mg
- Potassium (K): 347 mg
- Phosphorus: 241 mg

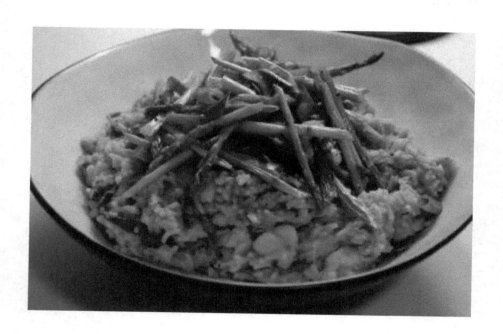

29. Sardine Fish Cakes

Preparation Time: 10 minutes

Cooking Time: 10 minutes

Servings: 4

Ingredients:

- 11 oz. of sardines, canned, drained
- 1/3 cup of shallot, chopped
- 1 teaspoon of chili flakes
- ½ teaspoon of salt
- 2 tablespoon of wheat flour, whole grain
- 1 egg, beaten
- 1 tablespoon of chives, chopped
- 1 teaspoon of olive oil
- 1 teaspoon of butter

Directions:

1. Put the butter in the skillet and melt it.
2. Add shallot and cook it until translucent.
3. After this, transfer the shallot to the mixing bowl.
4. Add sardines, chili flakes, salt, flour, egg, chives, and mix up until smooth with the help of the fork.
5. Make the medium size cakes and place them in the skillet.
6. Add olive oil.
7. Roast the fish cakes for 3 minutes from each side over medium heat.
8. Dry the cooked fish cakes with a paper towel if needed and transfer in the serving plates.

Nutrition:

- Calories: 221g
- Fat: 12.2g
- Fiber: 0.1g
- Carbs: 5.4g
- Protein: 21.3g

30.   Beef Bulgogi

Prep:

15 mins

Cook:

2 mins

Additional:

1 hr

Total:

1 hr 17 mins

Servings:

4

Yield:

1 pound flank steak

Ingredients

1 pound flank steak, thinly sliced
5 tablespoons soy sauce
¼ cup sriracha sauce
¼ cup chopped green onion
2 ½ tablespoons white sugar
2 tablespoons whole dried cayenne peppers
2 tablespoons minced garlic
2 tablespoons sesame seeds
2 tablespoons sesame oil
1 teaspoon ground cayenne pepper, or to taste
½ teaspoon ground black pepper

Directions
1
Place flank steak slices in a shallow dish.

2

Mix soy sauce, sriracha sauce, green onion, sugar, whole dried peppers, garlic, sesame seeds, sesame oil, ground cayenne, and black pepper together in a bowl. Pour over steak. Cover with plastic wrap and refrigerate to marinate, at least 1 hour but preferably overnight.

3

Preheat an outdoor grill for high heat, and lightly oil the grate.

4

Remove steak slices from marinade and grill on preheated grill until slightly charred and cooked through, 1 to 2 minutes per side.

5

Simmer marinade in a wok or skillet over medium heat until thick and the consistency of gravy; pour over grilled steak.

Nutritions
Per Serving: 248 calories; protein 16.3g; carbohydrates 15g; fat 13.8g; cholesterol 25.2mg; sodium 1792.2mg.

31.Zucchini Soup

Servings:

8

Yield:

8 servings

Ingredients

10 cups zucchini chunks
4 tablespoons margarine
2 large potatoes, peeled and chopped
1 onion, chopped
1 cup chicken broth
1 tablespoon chopped fresh tarragon
1 tablespoon dried savory
1 tablespoon fresh basil
1 tablespoon chopped fresh parsley
1 cup milk

Directions

1

Heat the butter in a large saucepan. Add the zucchini, potatoes and onion. Cover and cook for 2 minutes on high heat, shaking pan occasionally to prevent sticking on bottom.

2

Add chicken broth. Lower heat to medium low. Simmer until potatoes are tender, about 15 to 20 minutes.

3

Add the freshly chopped herbs and milk. Heat. Serve hot with a spoonful of sour cream on top of each serving.

Nutritions

Per Serving: 171 calories; protein 5.6g; carbohydrates 24.7g; fat 6.5g; cholesterol 2.4mg; sodium 192mg

Chapter 6. DESSERTS

32. Pineapple Protein Smoothie

Preparation Time: 10minutes

Cooking Time: 0 minutes

Servings: 1

Ingredients:

- 3/4 cup of pineapple sorbet
- 1 scoop of vanilla protein powder
- 1/2 cup of water
- 2 ice cubes, optional

Directions:

1. First, start by putting all the ingredients in a blender jug.
2. Give it a pulse for 30 seconds until blended well.
3. Serve chilled and fresh.

Nutrition:

- Calories: 268
- Protein: 18 g
- Fat: 4g
- Cholesterol: 36 mg
- Potassium: 237 mg
- Calcium: 160 mg
- Fiber: 1.4g

33.   Fruity Smoothie

Preparation Time: 10minutes

Cooking Time: 0 minutes

Servings: 2

Ingredients:

- 8 oz. of canned fruits, with juice
- 2 scoops of vanilla-flavored whey protein powder
- 1 cup of cold water
- 1 cup of crushed ice

Directions:

1. First, start by putting all the ingredients in a blender jug.
2. Give it a pulse for 30 seconds until blended well.
3. Serve chilled and fresh.

Nutrition:

- Calories 186
- Protein 23 g
- Fat 2g
- Cholesterol 41 mg
- Potassium 282 mg
- Calcium 160 mg
- Fiber 1.1 g

34. Mixed Berry Protein Smoothie

Preparation Time: 10minutes

Cooking Time: 0 minutes

Servings: 2

Ingredients:

- 4 oz. of cold water
- 1 cup of frozen mixed berries
- 2 ice cubes
- 1 tsp. of blueberry essence
- 1/2 cup of whipped cream topping
- 2 scoops of whey protein powder

Directions:

1. First, start by putting all the ingredients in a blender jug.
2. Give it a pulse for 30 seconds until blended well.
3. Serve chilled and fresh.

Nutrition:

- Calories 104
- Protein 6 g
- Fat 4 g
- Cholesterol 11 mg
- Potassium 141 mg
- Calcium 69 mg
- Fiber 2.4 g

35. Greek Cookies

Preparation Time: 20 minutes

Cooking Time: 25 minutes

Servings: 6

Ingredients:

- ½ cup of Plain yogurt
- ½ teaspoon of baking powder
- 2 tablespoons of Erythritol
- 1 teaspoon of almond extract
- ½ teaspoon of ground clove
- ½ teaspoon of orange zest, grated
- 3 tablespoons of walnuts, chopped
- 1 cup of wheat flour
- 1 teaspoon of butter, softened
- 1 tablespoon of honey
- 3 tablespoons of water

Directions:

1. In the mixing bowl, mix up together the plain yogurt, baking powder, Erythritol, almond extract, ground cloves, orange zest, flour, and butter.
2. Knead the non-sticky dough. Add olive oil if the dough is very sticky and knead it well.
3. Then make the log from the dough and cut it into small pieces.
4. Roll every piece of dough into the balls and transfer it in the lined baking paper tray.

5. Press the balls gently and bake for 25 minutes at 350F.

6. Meanwhile, heat up together honey and water. Simmer the liquid for 1 minute and remove from the heat.

7. When the cookies are cooked, remove them from the oven and let them cool for 5 minutes.

8. Then pour the cookies with sweet honey water and sprinkle with walnuts.

9. Cool the cookies.

Nutrition:

- Calories: 134
- Fat: 3.4
- Fiber: 0.9
- Carbs: 26.1
- Protein: 4.3

36.   Spiced Peaches

Servings:

24

Yield:

3 quarts

Ingredients

8 pounds peaches
1 cup sugar
4 cups water
2 cups honey
1 ½ teaspoons whole allspice
¾ teaspoon whole cloves
3 sticks cinnamon
3 Ball® or Kerr® Quart (32 oz) Jars with lids and bands

Directions

1

Prepare boiling water canner. Heat jars and lids in simmering water until ready to use. Do not boil. Set bands aside.

2

Wash, peel and pit peaches. Leave peaches in halves or cut into slices, if desired. Treat fruit to prevent browning.

3

Combine sugar, water and honey. Cook until sugar dissolves. Add peaches in syrup one layer at a time and cook for 3 minutes.

4

Pack hot peaches into hot jars leaving 1/2 inch headspace. Add 1/2 tsp allspice, 1/4 tsp cloves and 1 stick cinnamon to each jar.

5

Ladle hot syrup over peaches leaving 1/2 inch headspace. Remove air bubbles. Wipe rim. Center hot lid on jar. Apply band and adjust until fit is fingertip tight.

6

Process filled jars in a boiling water canner for 25 minutes, adjusting for altitude. Remove jars and cool. Check lids for seal after 24 hours. Lid should not flex up and down when center is pressed.

Nutritions
Per Serving: 148 calories; protein 0.1g; carbohydrates 38.9g; sodium 7.1mg.

37.   Chocolate Chip Cookies

Prep:

10 mins

Cook:

9 mins

Additional:

11 mins

Total:

30 mins

Servings:

30

Yield:

2 1/2 dozen

Ingredients

2 ¼ cups all-purpose flour
1 teaspoon baking soda
1 teaspoon salt
1 (3.3 ounce) package instant white chocolate pudding mix
1 cup butter, softened
1 cup white sugar
¾ cup brown sugar
2 eggs
2 teaspoons vanilla extract
2 cups semisweet chocolate chips

Directions

1

Preheat the oven to 375 degrees F (190 degrees C). Stir
together the flour, baking soda, salt and instant pudding
powder; set aside.

2

In a medium bowl, cream together the butter, white sugar and brown sugar until smooth. Blend in the eggs and vanilla. Gradually mix in the dry **Ingredients** until just blended. Stir in the chocolate chips by hand using a wooden spoon. Scoop cookies using an ice cream scoop or by heaping tablespoons. Place cookies at least 2 inches apart onto ungreased cookie sheets.

3

Bake for 8 to 10 minutes in the preheated oven, until lightly golden. Cool on baking sheets for a few minutes before removing to wire racks to cool completely.

Chapter 7. SMOOTHIES AND DRINKS

38.   Strawberry Fruit Smoothie

Preparation Time: 10minutes

Cooking Time: 0 minutes

Servings: 1

Ingredients:

- 3/4 cup of fresh strawberries
- 1/2 cup of liquid pasteurized egg whites
- 1/2 cup of ice
- 1 tbsp. of sugar

Directions:

1. First, start by putting all the ingredients in a blender jug.
2. Give it a pulse for 30 seconds until blended well.
3. Serve chilled and fresh.

Nutrition:

- Calories 156
- Protein 14 g
- Fat 0 g
- Cholesterol 0 mg
- Potassium 400 mg
- Phosphorus 49 mg

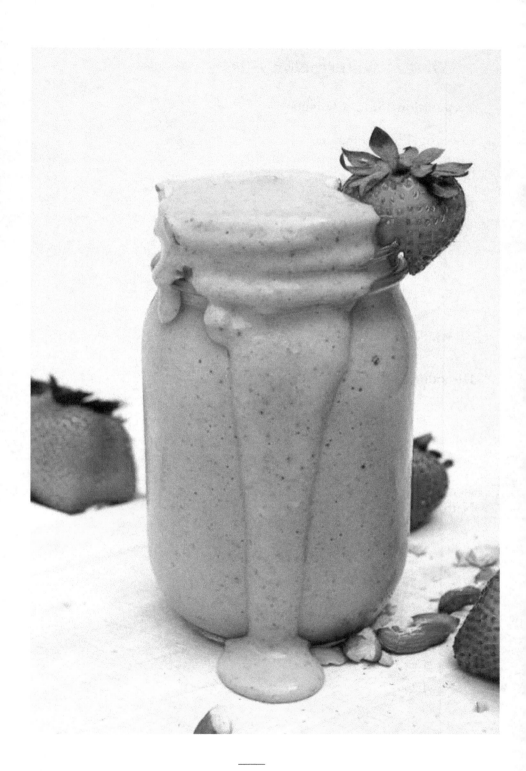

39.   Watermelon Bliss

Preparation Time: 10minutes

Cooking Time: 0 minutes

Servings: 2

Ingredients:

- 2 cups of watermelon
- 1 medium-sized cucumber, peeled and sliced
- 2 mint sprigs, leaves only
- 1 celery stalk
- Squeeze of lime juice

Directions:

1. First, start by putting all the ingredients in a blender jug.
2. Give it a pulse for 30 seconds until blended well.
3. Serve chilled and fresh.

Nutrition:

- Calories: 156
- Protein: 14 g
- Fat: 0 g
- Cholesterol: 0 mg
- Potassium: 400 mg
- Calcium: 29 mg
- Fiber: 2.5g

40. Cranberry Smoothie

Preparation Time: 10minutes

Cooking Time: 0 minutes

Servings: 1

Ingredients:

- 1 cup of frozen cranberries
- 1 medium cucumber, peeled and sliced
- 1 stalk of celery
- Handful of parsley
- Squeeze of lime juice

Directions:

1. First, start by putting all the ingredients in a blender jug. Give it a pulse for 30 seconds until blended well.
2. Serve chilled and fresh.

Nutrition:

- Calories: 126
- Protein: 12 g
- Fat: 0.03 g
- Cholesterol: 0 mg
- Potassium: 220 mg
- Calcium: 19 mg
- Fiber: 1.4g

41.Berry Cucumber Smoothie

Preparation Time: 10minutes

Cooking Time: 0 minutes

Servings: 1

Ingredients:

- 1 medium cucumber, peeled and sliced
- ½ cup of fresh blueberries
- ½ cup of fresh or frozen strawberries
- ½ cup of unsweetened rice milk
- Stevia, to taste

Directions:

1. First, start by putting all the ingredients in a blender jug.
2. Give it a pulse for 30 seconds until blended well.
3. Serve chilled and fresh.

Nutrition:

- Calories: 141
- Protein: 10 g
- Carbohydrates: 15 g
- Fat: 0 g
- Sodium: 113 mg
- Potassium: 230 mg
- Phosphorus: 129 mg

42.   Raspberry Peach Smoothie

Preparation Time: 10 minutes

Cooking Time: 0 minutes

Servings: 2

Ingredients:

- 1 cup of frozen raspberries
- 1 medium peach, pit removed, sliced
- ½ cup of silken tofu
- 1 tbsp. of honey
- 1 cup of unsweetened vanilla almond milk

Directions:

1. First, start by putting all the ingredients in a blender jug.
2. Give it a pulse for 30 seconds until blended well.
3. Serve chilled and fresh.

Nutrition:

- Calories: 132
- Protein: 9g
- Carbohydrates: 14 g
- Sodium: 112 mg
- Potassium: 310 mg
- Phosphorus: 39 mg
- Calcium: 32 mg

43.   Power-Boosting Smoothie

Preparation Time: 5 minutes

Cooking Time: 0 minutes

Servings: 2

Ingredients:

- ½ cup of water
- ½ cup of non-dairy whipped topping
- 2 scoops of whey protein powder
- 1½ cups of frozen blueberries

Directions:

1. In a high-speed blender, add all the ingredients and pulse until smooth.
2. Transfer into 2 serving glass and serve immediately.

Nutrition:

- Calories: 242
- Fat: 7g
- Carbs: 23.8g
- Protein: 23.2g
- Potassium (K): 263mg
- Sodium (Na): 63mg
- Phosphorous: 30 mg

44. Distinctive Pineapple Smoothie

Preparation Time: 5 minutes

Cooking Time: 0 minutes

Servings: 2

Ingredients:

- ¼ cup of crushed ice cubes
- 2 scoops of vanilla whey protein powder
- 1 cup of water
- 1½ cups of pineapple

Directions:

1. In a high-speed blender, add all the ingredients and pulse until smooth.
2. Transfer into 2 serving glass and serve immediately.

Nutrition:

- Calories: 117
- Fat: 2.1g
- Carbs: 18.2g
- Protein: 22.7g
- Potassium (K): 296mg
- Sodium (Na): 81mg
- Phosphorous: 28 mg

45. Pineapple Protein Smoothie

Preparation Time: 10minutes

Cooking Time: 0 minutes

Servings: 1

Ingredients:

- 3/4 cup of pineapple sorbet
- 1 scoop of vanilla protein powder
- 1/2 cup of water
- 2 ice cubes, optional

Directions:

4. First, start by putting all the ingredients in a blender jug.
5. Give it a pulse for 30 seconds until blended well.
6. Serve chilled and fresh.

Nutrition:

- Calories: 268
- Protein: 18 g
- Fat: 4g
- Cholesterol: 36 mg
- Potassium: 237 mg
- Calcium: 160 mg
- Fiber: 1.4g

46.   Fruity Smoothie

Preparation Time: 10minutes

Cooking Time: 0 minutes

Servings: 2

Ingredients:

- 8 oz. of canned fruits, with juice
- 2 scoops of vanilla-flavored whey protein powder
- 1 cup of cold water
- 1 cup of crushed ice

Directions:

4. First, start by putting all the ingredients in a blender jug.
5. Give it a pulse for 30 seconds until blended well.
6. Serve chilled and fresh.

Nutrition:

- Calories 186
- Protein 23 g
- Fat 2g
- Cholesterol 41 mg
- Potassium 282 mg
- Calcium 160 mg
- Fiber 1.1 g

47.   Mixed Berry Protein Smoothie

Preparation Time: 10minutes

Cooking Time: 0 minutes

Servings: 2

Ingredients:

- 4 oz. of cold water
- 1 cup of frozen mixed berries
- 2 ice cubes
- 1 tsp. of blueberry essence
- 1/2 cup of whipped cream topping
- 2 scoops of whey protein powder

Directions:

4. First, start by putting all the ingredients in a blender jug.
5. Give it a pulse for 30 seconds until blended well.
6. Serve chilled and fresh.

Nutrition:

- Calories 104
- Protein 6 g
- Fat 4 g
- Cholesterol 11 mg
- Potassium 141 mg
- Calcium 69 mg
- Fiber 2.4 g

48.   Peach High-Protein Smoothie

Preparation Time: 10minutes

Cooking Time: 0 minutes

Servings: 1

Ingredients:

- 1/2 cup of ice
- 2 tbsp. of powdered egg whites
- 3/4 cup of fresh peaches
- 1 tbsp. of sugar

Directions:

1. First, start by putting all the ingredients in a blender jug.
2. Give it a pulse for 30 seconds until blended well.
3. Serve chilled and fresh.

Nutrition:

- Calories 132
- Protein 10 g
- Fat 0 g
- Cholesterol 0 mg
- Potassium 353 mg
- Calcium 9 mg
- Fiber 1.9 g

49.   Strawberry Fruit Smoothie

Preparation Time: 10minutes

Cooking Time: 0 minutes

Servings: 1

Ingredients:

- 3/4 cup of fresh strawberries
- 1/2 cup of liquid pasteurized egg whites
- 1/2 cup of ice
- 1 tbsp. of sugar

Directions:

4. First, start by putting all the ingredients in a blender jug.
5. Give it a pulse for 30 seconds until blended well.
6. Serve chilled and fresh.

Nutrition:

- Calories 156
- Protein 14 g
- Fat 0 g
- Cholesterol 0 mg
- Potassium 400 mg
- Phosphorus 49 mg
- Calcium 29 mg
- Fiber 2.5 g

50.   Watermelon Bliss

Preparation Time: 10minutes

Cooking Time: 0 minutes

Servings: 2

Ingredients:

- 2 cups of watermelon
- 1 medium-sized cucumber, peeled and sliced
- 2 mint sprigs, leaves only
- 1 celery stalk
- Squeeze of lime juice

Directions:

4. First, start by putting all the ingredients in a blender jug.
5. Give it a pulse for 30 seconds until blended well.
6. Serve chilled and fresh.

Nutrition:

- Calories: 156
- Protein: 14 g
- Fat: 0 g
- Cholesterol: 0 mg
- Potassium: 400 mg
- Calcium: 29 mg
- Fiber: 2.5g

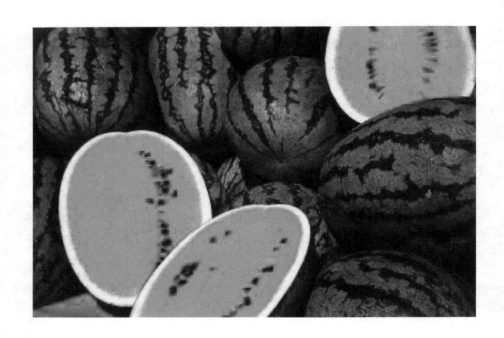

51. Cranberry Smoothie

Preparation Time: 10minutes

Cooking Time: 0 minutes

Servings: 1

Ingredients:

- 1 cup of frozen cranberries
- 1 medium cucumber, peeled and sliced
- 1 stalk of celery
- Handful of parsley
- Squeeze of lime juice

Directions:

3. First, start by putting all the ingredients in a blender jug. Give it a pulse for 30 seconds until blended well.
4. Serve chilled and fresh.

Nutrition:

- Calories: 126
- Protein: 12 g
- Fat: 0.03 g
- Cholesterol: 0 mg
- Potassium: 220 mg
- Calcium: 19 mg
- Fiber: 1.4g

52. Berry Cucumber Smoothie

Preparation Time: 10minutes

Cooking Time: 0 minutes

Servings: 1

Ingredients:

- 1 medium cucumber, peeled and sliced
- ½ cup of fresh blueberries
- ½ cup of fresh or frozen strawberries
- ½ cup of unsweetened rice milk
- Stevia, to taste

Directions:

4. First, start by putting all the ingredients in a blender jug.
5. Give it a pulse for 30 seconds until blended well.
6. Serve chilled and fresh.

Nutrition:

- Calories: 141
- Protein: 10 g
- Carbohydrates: 15 g
- Fat: 0 g
- Sodium: 113 mg
- Potassium: 230 mg
- Phosphorus: 129 mg

53.   Raspberry Peach Smoothie

Preparation Time: 10 minutes

Cooking Time: 0 minutes

Servings: 2

Ingredients:

- 1 cup of frozen raspberries
- 1 medium peach, pit removed, sliced
- ½ cup of silken tofu
- 1 tbsp. of honey
- 1 cup of unsweetened vanilla almond milk

Directions:

4. First, start by putting all the ingredients in a blender jug.
5. Give it a pulse for 30 seconds until blended well.
6. Serve chilled and fresh.

Nutrition:

- Calories: 132
- Protein: 9g
- Carbohydrates: 14 g
- Sodium: 112 mg
- Potassium: 310 mg
- Phosphorus: 39 mg
- Calcium: 32 mg

54.   Power-Boosting Smoothie

Preparation Time: 5 minutes

Cooking Time: 0 minutes

Servings: 2

Ingredients:

- ½ cup of water
- ½ cup of non-dairy whipped topping
- 2 scoops of whey protein powder
- 1½ cups of frozen blueberries

Directions:

3. In a high-speed blender, add all the ingredients and pulse until smooth.
4. Transfer into 2 serving glass and serve immediately.

Nutrition:

- Calories: 242
- Fat: 7g
- Carbs: 23.8g
- Protein: 23.2g
- Potassium (K): 263mg
- Sodium (Na): 63mg
- Phosphorous: 30 mg

55.   Distinctive Pineapple Smoothie

Preparation Time: 5 minutes

Cooking Time: 0 minutes

Servings: 2

Ingredients:

- ¼ cup of crushed ice cubes
- 2 scoops of vanilla whey protein powder
- 1 cup of water
- 1½ cups of pineapple

Directions:

3. In a high-speed blender, add all the ingredients and pulse until smooth.
4. Transfer into 2 serving glass and serve immediately.

Nutrition:

- Calories: 117
- Fat: 2.1g
- Carbs: 18.2g
- Protein: 22.7g
- Potassium (K): 296mg
- Sodium (Na): 81mg
- Phosphorous: 28 mg

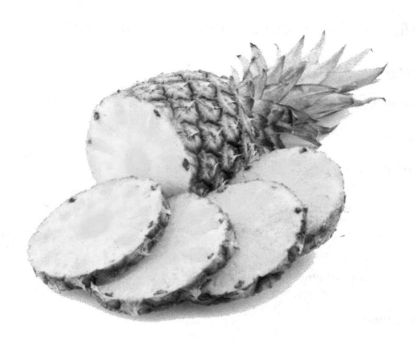

Chapter 8. SOUPS AND STEWS

56. Vegetable Lentil Soup

Preparation Time: 10 minutes

Cooking Time: 25 minutes

Servings: 4

Ingredients:

- 1 tablespoon of extra-virgin olive oil
- ½ sweet onion, diced
- 2 carrots, diced
- 2 celery stalks, diced
- ½ cup of lentils
- 5 cups of Simple Chicken Broth or low-sodium store-bought chicken stock
- 2 cups of sliced chard leaves
- Freshly ground black pepper
- Juice of 1 lemon

Directions:

1. In a medium stockpot over medium-high heat, heat the olive oil. Add the onion and stir until softened, about 3 to 5 minutes.
2. Add the carrots, celery, lentils, and broth. Bring to a boil, reduce the heat, and simmer, uncovered, for 15 minutes, until the lentils are tender.
3. Add the chard and cook for 3 additional minutes, until wilted.
4. Season it with pepper and lemon juice. Serve.

5. Substitution tip: you can use any greens that you have on hand for this soup; just adjust Cooking Times as needed based on the type. Collard, mustard, and turnip greens will need more Cooking Time, while spinach or bok choy will require just a couple of minutes, much like chard.

Nutrition:

- Calories: 186
- Total Fat: 11g
- Carbohydrates: 17g;
- Fiber: 3g
- Protein: 7g
- Phosphorus: 125mg
- Potassium: 557mg
- Sodium: 148mg

57.   Simple Chicken and Rice Soup

Preparation Time: 10 minutes

Cooking Time: 15 minutes

Servings: 4

Ingredients:

- 1 tablespoon of extra-virgin olive oil
- ½ sweet onion, chopped
- 2 celery stalks, chopped
- 2 carrots, chopped
- 8 ounces chicken breast, diced
- 4 cups of Simple Chicken Broth or low-sodium store-bought chicken stock
- ¼ teaspoon of dried thyme leaves
- 1 cup of cooked rice
- Juice of 1 lime
- Freshly ground black pepper
- 2 tablespoons of chopped parsley leaves, for garnish

Directions:

1. In a medium stockpot, heat the olive oil over medium-high heat. Add the onion, celery, carrots, and cook, often stirring, for about 5 minutes, until the onion begins to soften.
2. Add the chicken breast and continue stirring until the meat is just browned, but not cooked through. Add the broth and thyme, and bring to a boil. Reduce the heat and simmer for 10 minutes, until the chicken is cooked through and the vegetables are tender.

3. Add the rice and lime juice. Season it with pepper. Serve and garnished with parsley leaves.

4. Lower sodium tip: Choosing the Simple Chicken Broth over the store-bought variety will allow you better to control the amount of sodium in the finished product.

Nutrition:

- Calories: 176
- Total Fat: 11g
- Cholesterol: 26mg
- Carbohydrates: 17g
- Fiber: 3g
- Protein: 7g
- Phosphorus: 225mg
- Potassium: 357mg
- Sodium: 128mg

58.   Chicken Pho

Preparation Time: 10 minutes

Cooking Time: 15 minutes

Servings: 4

Ingredients:

- 5 cups of Simple Chicken Broth or low-sodium store-bought chicken stock
- 1-inch piece ginger cut lengthwise into 2 or 3 strips
- 1 cup of cooked chicken breast, diced
- Several fresh Thai basil sprigs
- 1 cup of mung bean sprouts
- 1 lime, cut into wedges
- 1 jalapeño pepper, stemmed, seeded, and thinly sliced
- 1 (16-ounce) package dried rice vermicelli noodles, cooked according to package Directions
- 4 tablespoons (¼ cups) of sliced scallions
- 4 tablespoons (¼ cups) of chopped cilantro leaves

Directions:

1. In a medium stockpot over medium-high heat, add the broth and ginger, and bring to a simmer. Add the chicken and simmer for 5 minutes. Remove the ginger from the pot and discard.
2. On a plate, arrange the Thai basil, bean sprouts, lime wedges, and jalapeño slices.

3. Distribute the noodles among four bowls. Add 1¼ cups of broth to each bowl. Top with 1 tablespoon each of the scallions and cilantro. Serve immediately, alongside the plate of garnishes.

4. Substitution tip: if you can't find fresh Thai basil near you, you can substitute regular basil, available in the fresh herb section of your grocery store.

Nutrition:

- Calories: 176
- Total Fat: 31g
- Cholesterol: 26mg
- Carbohydrates: 17g
- Fiber: 3g
- Protein: 7g
- Phosphorus: 225mg
- Potassium: 527mg
- Sodium: 138mg

59.   Turkey Burger Soup

Preparation Time: 10minutes

Cooking Time: 25 minutes

Servings: 4

Ingredients:

- 2 tablespoons of extra-virgin olive oil
- 1-pound of ground turkey breast
- ½ sweet onion, chopped
- 3 garlic cloves, minced
- Freshly ground black pepper
- 1 (16-ounce) can low-sodium diced tomatoes, drained
- 4 cups of Simple Chicken Broth or low-sodium store-bought chicken stock
- 1 cup of sliced carrots
- 1 cup of sliced celery
- 1 tablespoon of chopped fresh basil
- 1 tablespoon of chopped fresh oregano
- 1 tablespoon of chopped fresh thyme

Directions:

1. In a medium stockpot over medium-high heat, heat the olive oil. Add the turkey, onion, and garlic, and cook, stirring frequently, until the turkey is browned. Season it with pepper.
2. Add the drained tomatoes, broth, carrots, celery, basil, oregano, and thyme. Reduce the heat to low, and simmer for 20 minutes. Serve.

3. Substitution tip: if you don't have fresh basil, oregano, or thyme, use dried instead. Substitute 1 teaspoon of dried herbs for each tablespoon of fresh.

Nutrition:

- Calories: 186
- Fat: 11g
- Cholesterol: 26mg
- Carbohydrates: 17g
- Fiber: 3g
- Protein: 7g
- Phosphorus: 115mg
- Potassium: 257mg
- Sodium: 128mg

60. Turkey, Wild Rice, and Mushroom Soup

Preparation Time: 15 minutes

Cooking Time: 2-3 hours

Servings: 6

Ingredients:

- ½ cup of onion, chopped
- ½ cup of red bell pepper, chopped
- ½ cup of carrots, chopped
- 2 garlic cloves, minced
- 2 cup of cooked turkey, shredded
- 5 cup of chicken broth (see recipe)
- ½ cup of quick-cooking wild rice, uncooked
- 1 tbsp. of olive oil
- 1 cup of mushrooms, sliced
- 2 bay leaves
- ¼ tsp. of Mrs. Dash® Original salt-free herb seasoning blend
- 1 tsp. of dried thyme
- ½ tsp. of low sodium salt
- ¼ tsp. of black pepper

Directions:

1. Cook rice in a saucepan with 1-2 cups of broth. Set aside.
2. Heat the oil in a skillet and sauté the onion, bell pepper, carrots, and garlic until soft. Add to a 4 to 6-quart slow cooker.

3. Add remaining ingredients to the slow cooker except for the rice and mushrooms.
4. Cover and cook for 2-3 hours on LOW.
5. Add the mushrooms and rice and cook for a further 15 minutes.
6. Remove the bay leaves and serve.

Nutrition:

- Calories: 136
- Fat: 11g
- Cholesterol: 26mg
- Carbohydrates: 15g
- Fiber: 3g
- Protein: 5g
- Phosphorus: 145mg
- Potassium: 537mg
- Sodium: 128mg

Chapter 9. VEGETABLES

61.Zucchini Pasta with Mango-Kiwi Sauce

Preparation Time: 10 minutes

Cooking Time: 0 minutes

Servings: 2

Ingredients:

- 1 tsp. of dried herbs – optional
- ½ cup of Raw Kale leaves, shredded
- 2 small dried figs
- 3 medjool dates
- 4 medium kiwis
- 2 big mangos, peeled and seed discarded
- 2 cup of zucchini, spiralized
- ¼ cup of roasted cashew

Directions:

1. On a salad bowl, place kale, then topped with zucchini noodles and sprinkle with dried herbs. Set aside.
2. In a food processor, grind to a powder the cashews. Add figs, dates, kiwis, and mangoes, then puree to a smooth consistency.
3. Pour over zucchini pasta, serve and enjoy.

Nutrition:

- Calories: 370

- Fat: 9g
- Carbs: 76g
- Protein: 6g
- Fiber: 9g
- Sodium: 8mg
- Potassium: 868mg

62. Ratatouille

Preparation Time: 10 minutes

Cooking Time: 25 minutes

Servings: 4

Ingredients:

- Freshly ground black pepper
- ½ cup of shredded fresh basil leaves
- 1 tsp. of salt
- 4 plum tomatoes, coarsely chopped
- 1 red bell pepper, julienned
- 1 small zucchini, spiralized
- 1 small eggplant, spiralized
- 1 small bay leaf
- 4 garlic cloves, peeled and minced
- 1 onion, sliced thinly
- 1 tbsp. of olive oil

Directions:

1. Place a large nonstick saucepan on medium-slow fire and heat oil. Add bay leaf, garlic, and onion. Sauté until onions are translucent and soft. Add eggplant and cook for 7 minutes while occasionally stirring.
2. Add salt, tomatoes, red bell pepper, and zucchini, then increase the fire to medium-high. Continue cooking until veggies are tender, around 5 to 7 minutes.
3. Turn off fire and add pepper and basil. Stir to mix.
4. Serve and enjoy.

Nutrition:

- Calories: 116
- Fat: 4g
- Carbs: 21g
- Protein: 2g
- Fiber: 5g
- Sodium: 595mg
- Potassium: 421mg

63.   Roasted Eggplant with Feta Dip

Preparation Time: 10 minutes

Cooking Time: 30 minutes

Servings: 6

Ingredients:

- Pinch of sugar
- ¼ tsp. of salt
- ¼ tsp. of cayenne pepper or to taste
- 1 tbsp. of parsley, flat-leaf and chopped finely
- 2 tbsp. of fresh basil, chopped
- 1 small chili pepper, seeded and minced, optional
- ½ cup of red onion, finely chopped
- ½ cup of Greek feta cheese, crumbled
- ¼ cup of extra virgin olive oil
- 2 tbsp. of lemon juice
- Around 1 lb. of 1 medium eggplant

Directions:

1. Preheat broiler and position rack 6 inches away from heat source.
2. Pierce the eggplant with a knife or fork. Then with a foil, line a baking pan, place the eggplant, and broil. Make sure to turn eggplant every five minutes or until the skin is charred and eggplant is soft, which takes around 14 to 18 minutes of broiling. Once done, remove from heat and let cool.
3. In a medium bowl, add lemon. Then cut the eggplant in half, lengthwise, scrape the flesh, and place it in the bowl with lemon. Add

oil and mix until well combined. Then add salt, cayenne, parsley, basil, chili pepper, bell pepper, onion, and feta. Toss until well combined and add sugar to taste if wanted.

Nutrition:

- Calories: 139
- Fat: 12g
- Carbs: 7g
- Protein: 3g
- Fiber: 3g
- Sodium: 178mg
- Potassium: 249mg

64. Vegetable Potpie

Preparation Time: 10 minutes

Cooking Time: 10 minutes

Servings: 8

Ingredients:

- 1 recipe pastry for double-crust pie
- 2 tbsp. of cornstarch
- 1 tsp. of ground black pepper
- 1 tsp. of kosher salt
- 3 cups of vegetable broth
- 1 cup of fresh green beans, trimmed and snapped into ½ inch pieces
- 2 cups of cauliflower florets
- 2 stalks celery, sliced ¼ inch wide
- 2 potatoes, peeled and diced
- 2 large carrots, diced
- 1 clove garlic, minced
- 8 oz. of mushroom
- 1 onion, chopped
- 2 tbsp. of olive oil

Directions:

1. In a large saucepan, sauté garlic in oil until lightly browned, add onions and continue sautéing until soft and translucent.
2. Add celery, potatoes, carrots, and sauté for 3 minutes.

3. Add vegetable broth, green beans, cauliflower, and bring to a boil. Slow fire and simmer until vegetables are slightly tender. Season it with pepper and salt.

4. Mix ¼ cup water and cornstarch in a small bowl. Stir until the mixture is smooth and has no lumps. Then pour into the vegetable pot while mixing constantly.

5. Continue mixing until soup thickens, around 3 minutes. Remove from fire.

6. Meanwhile, roll out pastry dough and place on an oven-safe 11x7 baking dish. Pour the vegetable filling and then cover with another pastry dough. Seal and flute the edges of the dough and prick the top dough with a fork in several places.

7. Bake the dish in a preheated oven of 425 °F for 30 minutes or until crust has turned a golden brown.

Nutrition:

- Calories: 202
- Fat: 10g
- Carbs: 26g
- Protein: 4g
- Fiber: 3g
- Sodium: 466mg
- Potassium: 483mg

65. Marsala Roasted Carrots

Preparation Time: 10 minutes

Cooking Time: 40 minutes

Servings: 8

Ingredients:

- Chopped fresh parsley – optional
- Pepper and salt to taste
- 2 tbsp. of balsamic vinegar
- 2 tbsp. of extra virgin olive oil
- ½ cup of marsala
- 2 lbs. of julienned carrots

Directions:

1. Peel and julienne the carrots
2. Place carrots on the baking sheet.
3. Add vinegar, olive oil, and Marsala. Toss to coat.
4. Roast carrots in the oven for 30 minutes at 425oF, while occasionally stirring.
5. Carrots are cooked once tender and lightly browned. Remove from oven and season it with pepper, salt, and fresh parsley.

Nutrition:

- Calories: 62
- Fat: 2g
- Carbs: 11g
- Protein: 1g

CPSIA information can be obtained
at www.ICGtesting.com
Printed in the USA
BVHW092156080621
609009BV00008B/755